TEDDY GETS A FILLING

Authored by
Elizabeth Mahadeo RDH

Illustrated by
Alexandra Barth

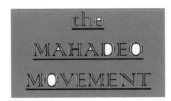

the
MAHADEO
MOVEMENT

Published by the Mahadeo Movement

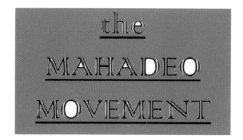

First Edition Copyright© 2012 by Elizabeth Mahadeo

createspace.com/3900582   amazon.com/author/elizabethmahadeo   emahadeo.wordpress.com
facebook.com/TheMahadeoMovement   @mahadeoE

ISBN 978-0956943828

I dedicate this story to children and their healthy, beautiful smiles.

For parents- Although it can be tempting not to fix primary (baby) teeth for a variety of reasons, it is necessary to take care of these teeth. Primary teeth provide a path for permanent (adult) teeth to follow into proper alignment. The health or lack of health of a primary tooth can affect the health of the permanent teeth developing under the gums. Primary teeth are vital to your child's speech development and overall growth and development.

A nice smile is something a child can be proud of. Preventative appointments at the dental office, daily home care of teeth and gums, and fixing teeth when required lays the foundation for a child to value their oral health and total body health. Please consider this if your child needs dental treatment.

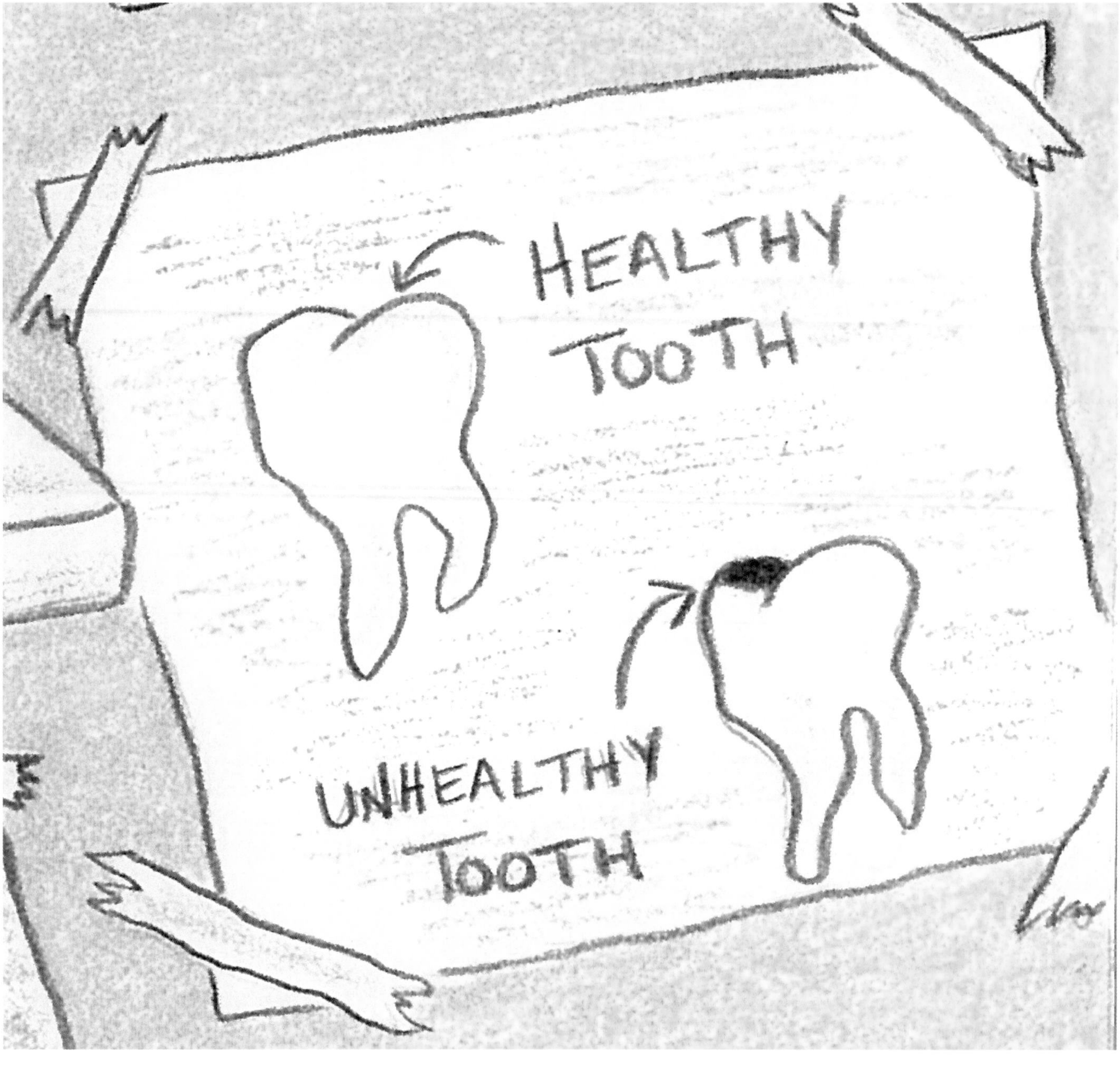
HEALTHY TOOTH
UNHEALTHY TOOTH

Teddy has a cavity in his tooth. A cavity happens when a tooth is decayed, meaning part of the enamel (and maybe the dentin) is sick from too many sugar bugs.

Sugar bugs are bad germs which make your teeth and gums unhealthy. The way to fix a cavity is to have a filling done at the dental office.

Teddy waits patiently in the reception area of the dental office for his appointment to see Dr. Dentin.

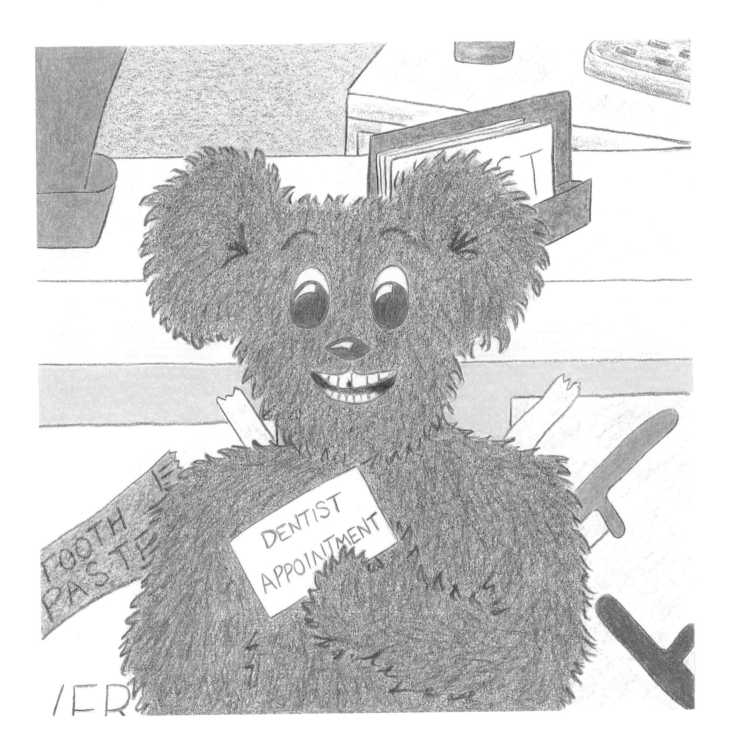

When it is his turn, Dr. Dentin's assistant comes to get Teddy from the reception area. He follows her back to the operatory.

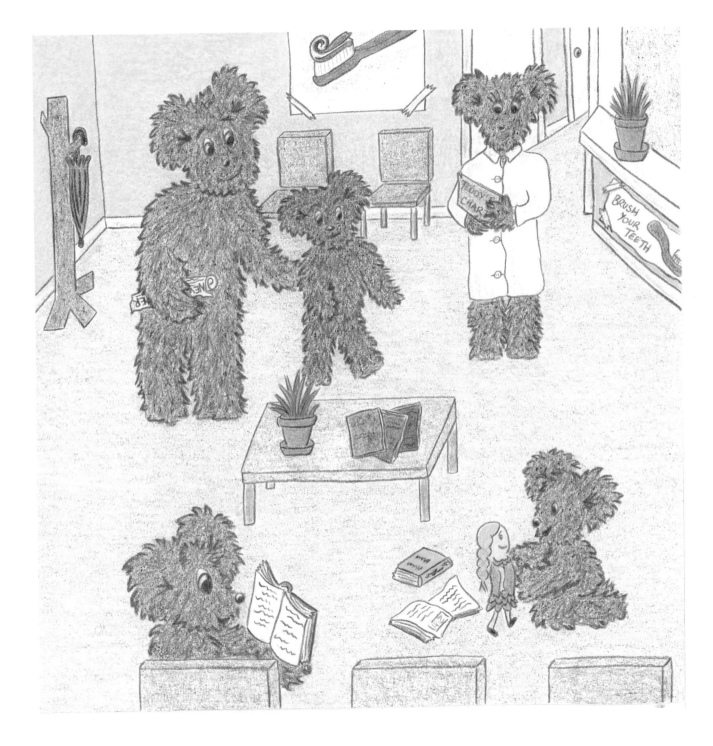

Teddy sits in the big comfy chair. The chair moves backwards until Teddy is laying down flat on his back.

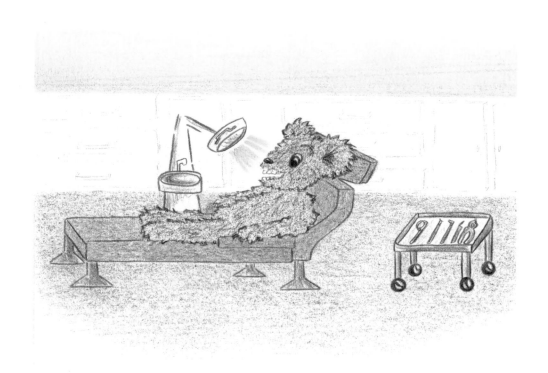

Dr. Dentin turns on the bright light and shines it into Teddy's mouth. The tooth counter and tiny mirror are ready for him to check Teddy's tooth.

Before Dr. Dentin fixes the sick tooth, he helps it fall asleep. It will sleep during the appointment and will stay asleep until after the filling is finished.

Dr. Dentin puts flavoured gel on Teddy's gums, making his gums numb in the area where the sick tooth is.

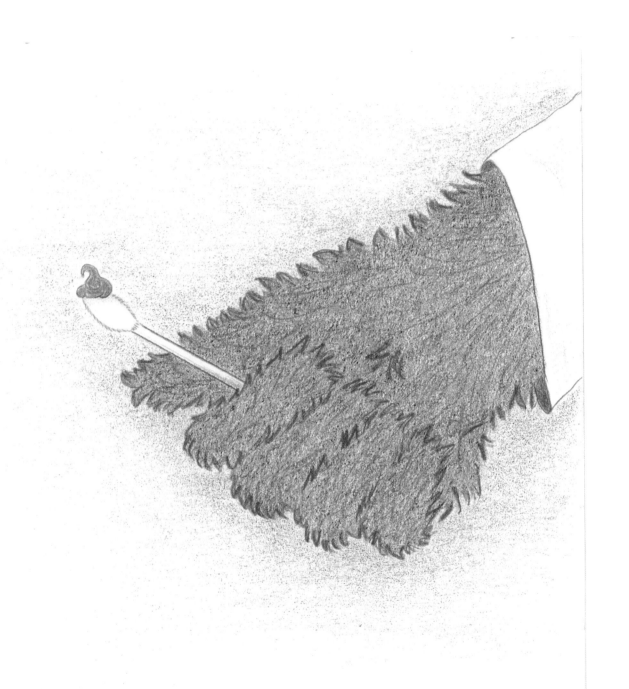

Dr. Dentin uses sleepy juice in a squirter to help Teddy's sick tooth fall asleep. The sleepy juice soaks into Teddy's gums and into the roots of his tooth. Now his tooth feels numb and sleepy.

It is ok to feel this way. Sometimes sleepy juice can make your lips feel big, but they aren't- ask to look in the mirror!

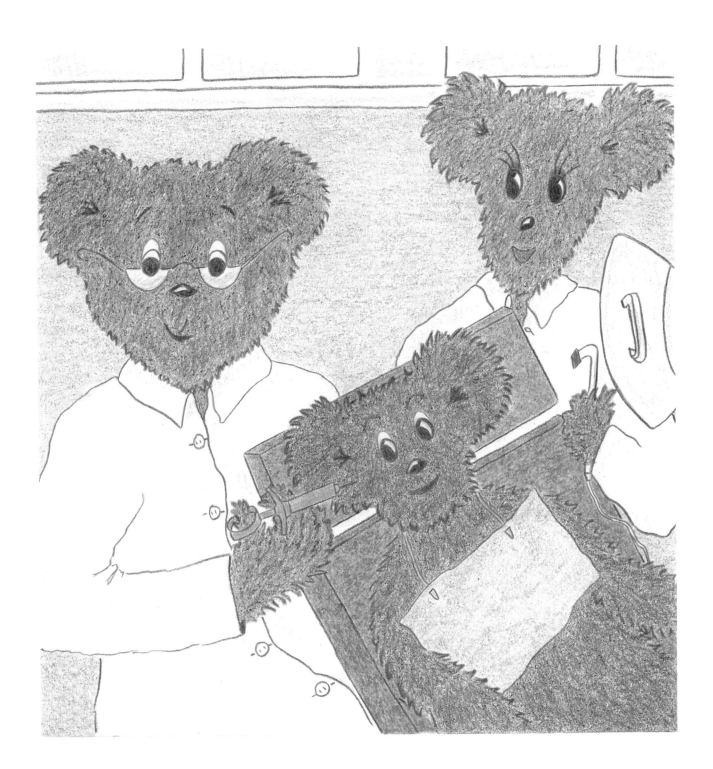

Dr. Dentin uses a special tool called the whistle to clean away the cavity. It is called the whistle because it sounds like a whistle!

Most of the sugar bugs are washed away with the water it sprays.

Dr. Dentin and his assistant use the vacuum to suck up the water, the sugar bugs, and some of Teddy's saliva. The vacuum makes a funny noise!

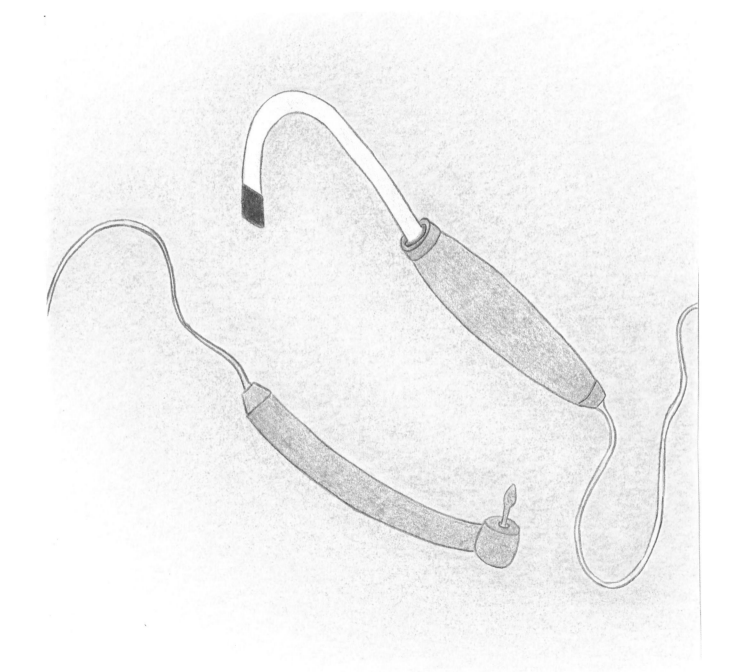

The sick part of the enamel and dentin has been cleaned away. What's left is a healthy tooth with a hole in it. Dr. Dentin must fill up the hole to make it a whole tooth again.

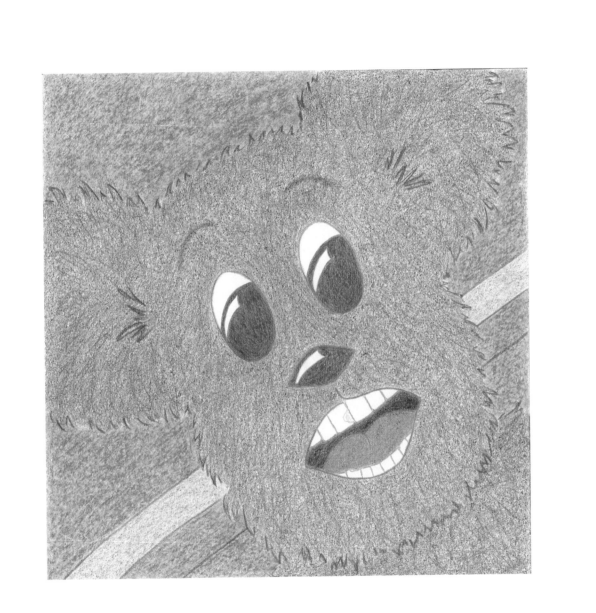

Dr. Dentin uses a special blue soap where the cavity used to be. This soap is a cleaner that makes sure all the sugar bugs are gone. Dr. Dentin and his assistant wash off the soap with a spray of water and the vacuum.

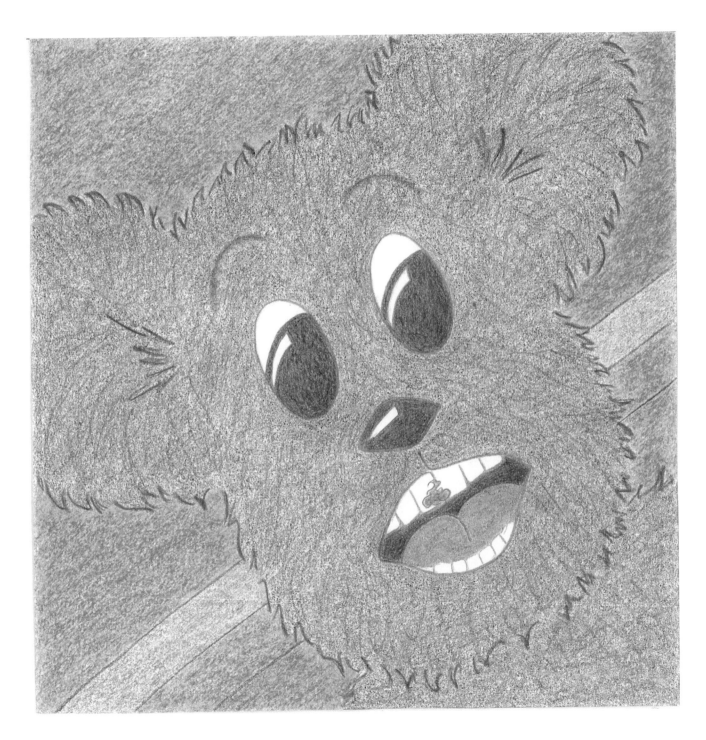

Dr. Dentin brushes clear glue onto Teddy's tooth.

Next he puts a white filling into the hole. At first the white filling is soft like dough. Dr. Dentin molds it into the proper shape of a whole tooth.

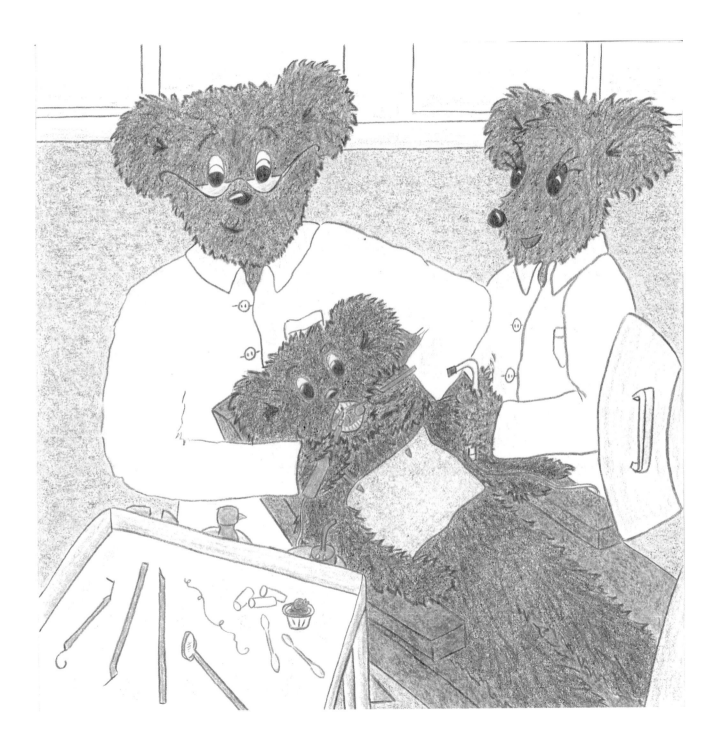

When the magic blue flashlight shines on the filling it magically turns hard.

Be careful not to look at the magic blue flashlight while it is shining, it is super bright!

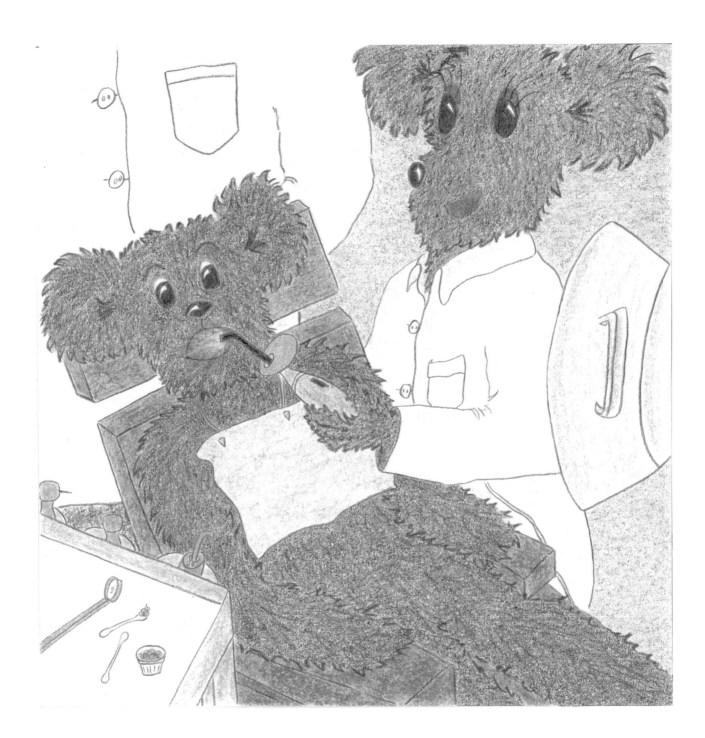

Dr. Dentin polishes the filling to make it smooth.   Next he checks the filling with special colourful paper to make sure Teddy's teeth bite together the right way.

Teddy's tooth is the same colour and shape as it was before it got sick. His tooth is healthy again!

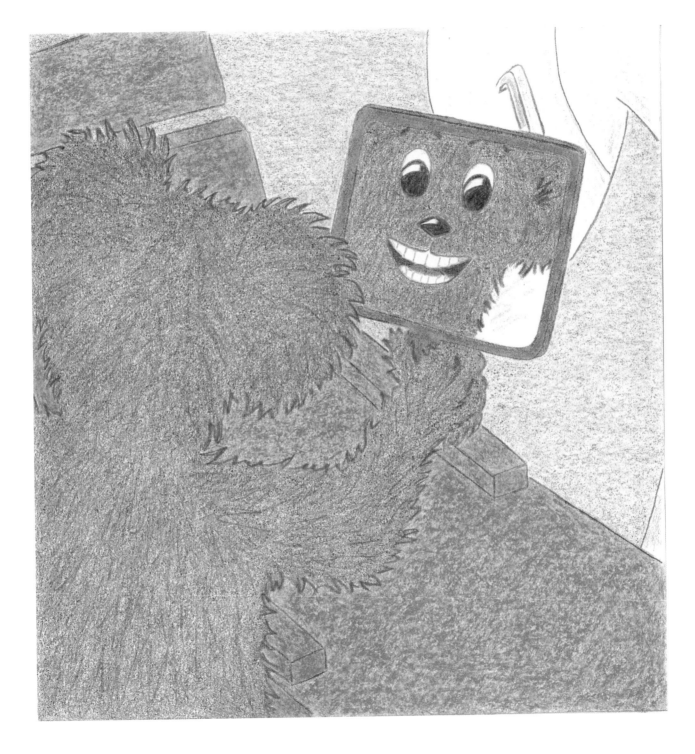

Dr. Dentin teaches Teddy how to fight against cavities. To do this, Teddy must remove all the plaque and sugar bugs from around his teeth and gums by flossing and brushing.

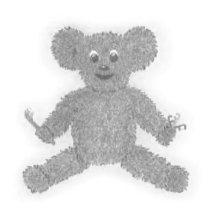

Flossing and brushing will keep Teddy's gums healthy, his teeth strong, and his body healthy.

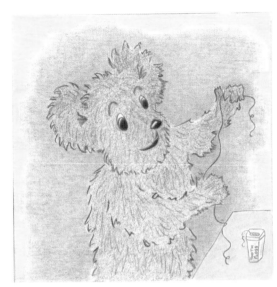

Teddy should floss at least once a day and brush before school in the morning, before bed at night, plus any other time in between!

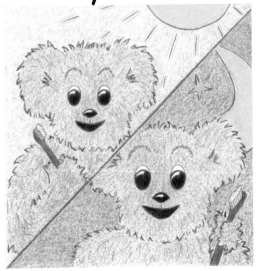

In a few hours Teddy's tooth will get tingly and wake up. It will feel just the way it did before falling asleep.

Teddy is careful not to bite his lips or cheeks or tongue while they are sleeping.

Teddy did so well at his dental appointment that he got a prize!

Good Job Teddy!

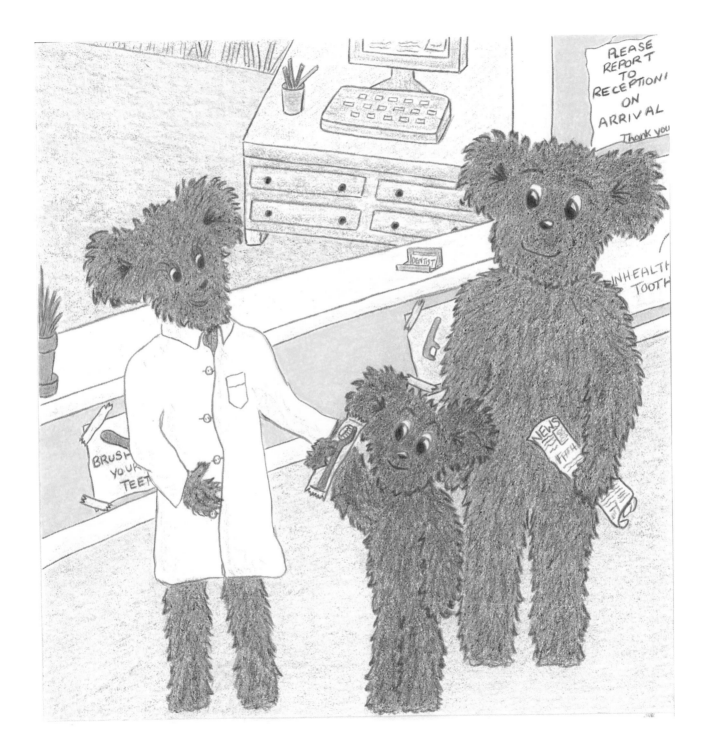

GLOSSARY

Air Water Syringe- sprays out water, sprays out air, and can spray out water and air at the same time! Ask to see it in action!

Anesthetic-is sleepy juice. It soaks into your gums and into the roots of your teeth. Sleepy juice makes your tooth numb.

Appointment- a special time just for you

Articulating Paper- colourful paper you bite your teeth on to check that the filling is just the right size and shape for you

Bond- clear glue used to prepare tooth for the filling

Calculus- hard plaque on teeth that can only be cleaned off with special tools at the dental office

Cavity- the decayed part of a tooth

Checkup- your special time when the Dentist and Dental Hygienist look at and feel your teeth to make sure they are healthy

Chewing Surface- the bumpy surface of your tooth that you eat with, where the food gets stuck

Cleaning- all the sugar bugs are washed away from your teeth and gums using special tooth tools

Decay- when a tooth or part of a tooth is sick from too many sugar bugs

Dental Hygienist- a person whose job it is to count, clean and check your teeth and gums

Dental Office- the place you go to have your appointment, where the Dentist and Dental Hygienist work

Dentin- the layer of tooth underneath the enamel

Dentist- a person whose job it is to check your teeth and gums, and who will fix your teeth if they need to be fixed

Enamel- the layer of tooth you see when you smile, it is hard and strong

Etch- a special blue soap used to clean a tooth after decay is removed to be to make sure all the sugar bugs are gone

Filling- when a tooth that is sick with too many sugar bugs is fixed. The cavity is cleaned away and the hole left behind in the tooth is filled up with a white, plastic filling material that looks and feels just like a real tooth

Floss- special string which slides between your teeth to clean away sugar bugs and plaque

Fluoride- a liquid or foam which goes on your teeth after they have been cleaned to make your teeth super strong to fight against cavities

Instruments- at the dental office, instruments are the tools used to count, check, clean, and fix your teeth

Magic Blue Flashlight- also called a curing light, it shines a bright blue light and makes the soft, white filling material very, very hard

Mirror- a mirror small enough to fit inside your mouth helps the dentist and dental hygienist see the back, sides, front and chewing surfaces of each tooth

Molars- the big teeth at the back of your mouth that you chew with

Numb- the sensation of not being able to feel your tooth

Operatory- a special room with special tools at the dental office, where your teeth get counted, checked, cleaned and fixed

Plaque- too many sugar bugs! Makes your teeth feel sticky and fuzzy

Polisher- a special toothbrush you only find at the dental office, it spins and gets your teeth very clean and shiny, is also used to polish fillings

Reception area- a room at the dental office that has books, magazines, toys and sometimes a TV, you stay there until it is your turn

Restoration- a technical term for a filling

Saliva- the watery stuff inside your mouth

Sleepy Juice- special liquid that helps your tooth go to sleep so it feels numb

Sleepy Juice Squirter- a holder for sleepy juice that helps the dentist squirt sleepy juice around your gums and teeth

Sugar bugs- bad germs that make your teeth and gums sick

Tooth Counter- also called an explorer, this instrument gently counts and checks your teeth

Toothpaste- gooey soap just for teeth

Vacuum- just like the one at home! It makes a sucking noise and slurrrps up your saliva

Whistle- also called a handpiece, it's a special tool which removes decay from a sick tooth

Happy Air

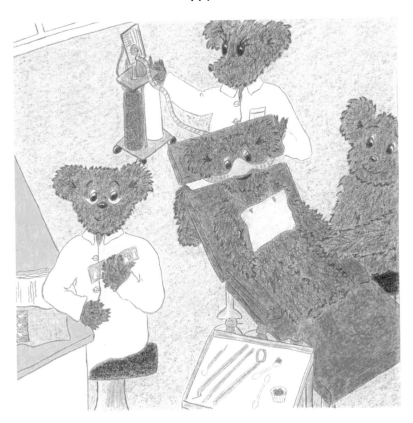

Sometimes the dentist will give you special air to breath during your appointment. This special air is called Nitrous Oxide, or happy air!

The dentist gives you a happy nose to wear over your own nose. You breathe in the special air from the happy nose and it makes you feel relaxed, good and happy!

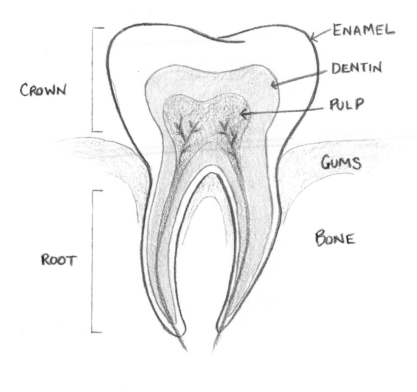

ENAMEL

DENTIN

PULP

CROWN

GUMS

BONE

ROOT

TOOTH LAYERS

(Torres et al., 1995, p. 61)

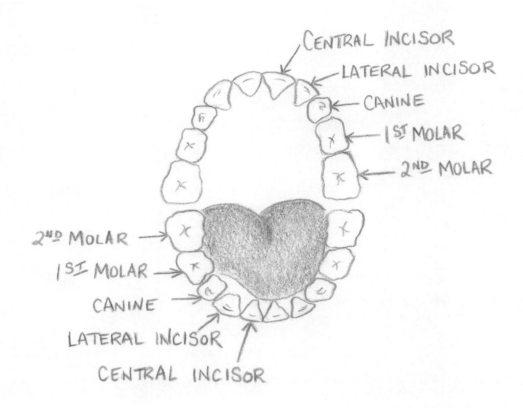

CENTRAL INCISOR

LATERAL INCISOR

CANINE

1ST MOLAR

2ND MOLAR

2ND MOLAR

1ST MOLAR

CANINE

LATERAL INCISOR

CENTRAL INCISOR

CHILDREN'S TEETH

(Torres et al., 1995, p. 59)

Normal Exfoliation and Eruption Patterns for Primary Teeth:

Upper Teeth	Eruption Date	Shedding Date
Central Incisors	8-12 months	6-7 years
Lateral Incisors	9-13 months	7-8 years
Canines	16-22 months	10-12 years
1st Molars	13-19 months	9-11 years
2nd Molars	25-33 months	10-12 years

Lower Teeth		
2nd Molars	23-31 months	10-12 years
1st Molars	14-18 months	9-11 years
Canines	17-23 months	9-12 years
Lateral Incisors	10-16 months	7-8 years
Central Incisors	6-10 months	6-7 years

(Torres et al, pg 59)

Normal Eruption Patterns for Permanent Teeth:

Upper Teeth	Eruption Date
Central Incisors	7-8 years
Lateral Incisors	8-9 years
Canines	11-12 years
1st Premolars	10-11 years
2nd Premolars	10-12 years
1st Molars	6-7 years
2nd Molars	12-13 years
3rd Molars	17-21 years

Lower Teeth	
3rd Molars	17-21 years
2nd Molars	11-13 years
1st Molars	6-7 years
2nd Premolars	11-12 years
1st Premolars	10-12 years
Canines	9-10 years
Lateral Incisors	7-8 years
Central Incisors	6-7 years

(Torres et all, pg 60)

References

Elizabeth Mahadeo RDH (nee Butler) attended George Brown College in Toronto, Canada. Her Certificate in Dental Assisting Levels I & II and Diploma in Dental Hygiene combined with many years of clinical experience have inspired her to write confidently on this topic. Her references include, but are not limited to:

Daniel, S.J., Harft, S.A. (2002). Mosby's Dental Hygiene: Concepts, Cases, and Competencies. St. Louis: Mosby Inc.

Darby, Michele L., Walsh, Margaret M. (2010). Dental Hygiene Theory and Practice Third Edition. St. Louis: Saunders Elsevier.

Torres, H.O., Ehrlich, A., Bird, D., Dietz, E. (1995). Modern Dental Assisting Fifth Edition. Philadelphia: W.B. Saunders Company.

Wilkins, E.M. (1999). Clinical Practice of the Dental Hygienist Eighth Edition. Philadelphia: Lippincott, Williams and Wilkins.

COMING SOON...

TEDDY TALKS
PREVENTION

Made in the USA
Charleston, SC
07 January 2013